The Professional Makeup Artist's Discount Guide

Never Pay Full Price
For Your Makeup Again

Toni Thomas

DEDICATION

Success is about dedication. You may not be where you
want to be or do what you want to do when you're on the
journey. But you've got to be willing to have vision and
foresight that leads you to an incredible end.

-Usher

CONTENTS

ACKNOWLEDGMENTS

I want to acknowledge every cosmetic company listed in this book who generously allow professional makeup artists to purchase their products at a discounted rate. Without their support and contributions to the beauty industry we would just be artists without mediums.

REQUIREMENT(S)

Putting together a professional makeup kit separate from your personal makeup kit will take effort, time, and money but utilizing the pro artist discount programs offered to you from some of your favorite cosmetic companies will help you build your pro kit at almost half the cost. Your professional makeup kit is your calling card and an essential tool of a professional makeup artist, so filling your kit with quality professional makeup is critical to your success. If you are planning to jump right into your career, you will need to start building your kit immediately and utilize the discounts offered to you at a fraction of the retail cost.

Purchasing quality products for your kit will be entirely up to you and the products you choose to use on your clients will also be up to you, so finding the best products for the best price is a smart move in your business. Most cosmetic companies know that professional grade products are expected in a professional makeup artists' kit and most companies will give you every opportunity to try these products at a discounted rate as well as purchase them for your kit below retail cost. The benefit for them is utilizing you the professional makeup artist as their best marketing tool. You will often be asked what products you use in your kit and in many cases, you will share your favorite products with your clients and rave about the benefits. If you are good at what you do you should be sharing with your clients what products you are using and how they should be applied. As a pro makeup artist you will love different products from different brands, but in every case, you will be expected to use professional grade products.

When building your pro kit be strategic and think about the essential products you need or the products that you will use most often. Think about your makeup bag and how it will be set up to give you the best layout for utilizing space and weight. Your makeup kit can get very heavy if you put too many unnecessary items within. This is often the case for new makeup artists who think they need to bring one of everything. Think about things that can double and be used for other applications. You don't need five shadow palettes if you can combine it down to three that will be universal for every application that is requested. Most makeup artists realize quickly that less is more and that many products are universal. Also if you are a bridal makeup artist who also does stylized makeup or special effects makeup you might want to have two separate kits. Either way, it will be up to you the professional makeup artist to get your bag set up with the best products utilizing good organization skills and getting the best products in your kit for flawless results on your clients.

When putting together the contents of your pro kit you will want to think about the tools you will need as well as the products you will use. Your tools are an extension of your hands and without a doubt an essential part of getting the best possible results for your clients. Using high-quality tools that weigh less and produce the best possible results are what you want to keep in mind as you build your kit. Many makeup artist tool manufacturers also offer pro discounts and pro artist programs. It will be up to you to do your research and find the best tools on the market and apply for their artist program if offered. Double ended brushes are a great way to get the best bang for your buck as well as providing you less weight in your case and more room to organize your makeup kit.

Many of your clients will look at your kit as a reflection of you, and you are a reflection of your business, and building a credible business should be your most important marketing strategy. The effort involved in applying for and keeping up on all the pro artist programs offered to you the professional will ultimately take time and energy, but the result will be a kit filled with pro products at a fraction of the retail cost. Take the time and the effort and organize your pro cards or pro accounts onto a journal or online note storage so you can easily access your credentials.

Please note as of the date of publication of this book the cosmetic companies listed in this directory currently have active pro artist programs. These programs are subject to change at any time.

What if you don't have a formal education and the requirements for your pro artist program with a cosmetic company call for a certificate or documentation of a formal education?

We recommend seeking out your local cosmetology programs or esthetic programs to see if they offer a professional makeup course. If you are unable to find a local class that teaches hands-on, then take the time to research online programs that provide Professional Makeup Courses designed with lesson plans, video tutorials, and have educational materials for you to utilize. These courses usually offer a certificate of completion that you can use as documentation for your requested credentials.

Here is a list of a few online schools that offer online Professional Makeup Artistry Courses.

Women in Gear: School of Makeup Artistry
www.womeningear.com

QC Makeup Academy
https://www.qcmakeupacademy.com

AOFM Makeup Academy
https://www.aofmakeup.com/online-makeup-school/

Academy of Glam
https://academyofglam.com

Makeup.School
https://makeup.school

M.A.C COSMETICS & BOBBI BROWN

MAC Cosmetics
www.maccosmetics.com

One of the industry's leading discount programs for the makeup professional, and for aspiring makeup artists getting an education in professional makeup artistry, esthetics, or cosmetology, is the MAC pro artist membership program. To enroll in their program, simply go online to MAC cosmetics, fill out the MAC Pro Artist Membership application and provide professional documentation (current and within one year) and membership fee. If you are accepted you will receive your card in a few weeks and can begin enjoying your membership benefits. You will receive reminders to renew. Every time your card expires and you will need to re-submit current professional documentation, the membership fee, and a completed MAC Pro Membership application. MAC Pro reserves the right to request additional professional documentation at any time.

An example of professional identification must be included with the application. Examples of professional identification include one of the following:

- union card
- professional license or publication masthead
- agency branded composite card
- editorial page with your name credit
- program or press material with name and profession
- professional website (must list profession and be self-hosted)
- certificate/diploma

Required professional identification must be current (within one year) and indicate your name and specific profession.

For those applying to the MAC Pro Student program, documentation can be a receipt, confirmation of class, program payment, a confirmation of class schedule. All documents must include first and last name, school name, program name, and start and end dates.

If you are a student, select the "Student" option from the professional drop down menu.

MAC Pro reserves the right to require additional professional documentation at any time. All professional documentation will be saved in your digital profile and not visible to anyone other than our customer service team. MAC Pro reserves the right to reject the application for any reason.

Bobbi Brown Cosmetics

www.bobbibrowncosmetics.com

The Bobbi Brown Pro card requirements are:

- One valid photo identification
- A Completed application

AND

Two pieces of the following professional makeup artist criteria (valid within the past two years):

- Composite Card
- Business card with name and specific Makeup Artist profession
- Editorial page with a name credit
- Union card
- Professional valid license
- Crew Call list on production company letterhead
- Reference letter from employer

Bobbi Brown Pro reserves the right to require additional professional documentation at any time. All professional documentation will be saved in your digital profile and not visible to anyone other than their pro artist customer service team. Bobbi Brown Pro reserves the right to reject the application for any reason.

THE DIRECTORY
A to Z

Here is a comprehensive list of cosmetic companies who give pro discounts to makeup artists and aspiring makeup artists at below retail prices. Most of the companies listed in this directory have a 20% to 40% discount and some even have up to 50% off the retail prices.

Applying online to all of these companies will take time and each company has the discretion to deny your application but if you want to build your pro kit this is where you will want to start.

Please note as of the date of publication the cosmetic companies listed in this directory currently have active pro artist programs. These programs are subject to change at any time.

It is your responsibility to follow all the pro artist guidelines listed for each company and always follow the industries professional code of conduct. Integrity in this business is everything!

18.21 Man Made

https://camerareadycosmetics.com/collections/18-21-man-made

Requirement(s): Apply and Refer to Camera Ready Cosmetics guidelines listed below.

Afterglow Cosmetics
www.afterglowcosmetics.com

Requirement(s): You will need to email your required documents email to artist@afterglowcosmetics.com

Two of the following will be accepted:

- A copy of your Union Card,
- TV or film crew list with name credit.
- Agency Confirmation – your representing agency can fax a roster list on the Agency's letter head with your name on the roster. The letter must include the Agency's contact information and website.
- State Esthetician or Makeup Artist Certificate

All professional discount orders must be placed over the phone by calling 866.630.4569.

Anastasia Beverly Hills
www.anastasiabeverlyhills.com

Their pro artist program has not launched yet but the website says, "coming soon."

Annabelle

https://www.annabelle.com/en_ca/

Requirement(s): To apply for this discount, they invite you to subscribe by sending your request to the following email address: prodiscount@groupemarcelle.com.

Subsequently, they will send you a membership application to complete and send us back by email along with a photo ID and proof of your profession. You will need to provide any two of proof of the items listed below. Here are some examples of attachments:

- Business card with name and mention of the profession
- Editorial Page with name credit
- Proof of agency representation
- Magazine tear sheet with name credit

Following receipt of this information, all requests will be evaluated and if your application is accepted, you will receive a code that you will use when shopping online.

The program membership will be valid for one year, from January 1 to December 31, and will be renewable upon request.

Artis Brushes

https://artisbrush.com/pages/artis-pro-program

Requirement(s): Provide copies of two of the following along with photo identification:

• Magazine tear sheet with name credit

• Program or call sheet

• Comp Card

• Union membership card

• Proof of agency representation (letter from agent or

link to roster)
• Website (gallery-sites or Facebook not valid)
• Blank Contract
• IMDb Credit
Name credit: document must state makeup artist's legal name.

Ardell Lashes
https://camerareadycosmetics.com/collections/ardell-lashes

Requirement(s) Apply and refer to Camera Ready Cosmetics pro artist guidelines.

BB Cosmetics & Makeup Online
http://www.bbmakeuponline.com/artist-programs

Requirement(s): A copy of Photo Identification and two pieces of Professional Criteria:
- Composite Card
- Business Card with name and specific profession
- Editorial Page with name credit
- Union Card
- Professional License
- Diploma/Certificate
- Publication Masthead
- Program/press Materials with name
- Contract on Production Company Letterhead
- Crew/Call List on Prod. Co. Letterhead
- Professional Letter of Reference of Employment

Send application to processing department at:

BB makeup cosmetic bar
Attn: BB pro membership
511 2nd St
Hudson, WI 54016
Barbara Mordini
https://bmartistlashes.com.au/professional-discount-application/

Requirement(s) To apply for an industry discount click on the professional industry link that best describes your business, and submit your online application.

Bdellium Tools
https://www.bdelliumtools.com/pages/bdellium-tools-pro

Requirement(s): Submit an application form, copy of a government/state photo ID, & 2 of the following:

- Makeup artist license
- Composite card
- Union card
- Professional website
- Reference letter from current employer
- Editorial page including name credit (highlight your name)
- Crew call list on production company letterhead (highlight your name)
- Program material with name (highlight your name)
- Submit application

Beaute Cosmetics
media@beaute-cosmetics.com

Requirement(s): To apply you must be a working makeup artist or industry professional, send a professional email to the address listed above to be considered for their pro artist program. contact media@beaute-cosmetics.com

Beauty Blender
https://camerareadycosmetics.com/collections/beautyblender

Requirement(s): Apply and refer to Camera Ready Cosmetics pro artist guidelines.

Becca Cosmetics
https://camerareadycosmetics.com/collections/becca

Requirement(s): Apply and Refer to Camera Ready Cosmetics guidelines.

Bella Pierre
https://www.bellapierre.com

I was unable to locate any pro makeup artist discount on the Bella Pierre website.

Ben Nye
https://camerareadycosmetics.com/collections/ben-nye

Requirement(s): Apply and Refer to Camera Ready Cosmetics guidelines.

Benefits San Francisco
https://pro.benefitcosmetics.com/us/

Requirement(s): Apply online: Submit one of the following:

- Union Card
- Professional License
- Publication Mast Head

Or two of the following:

- Comp Card
- Business card
- Editorial Page
- Contract
- Press Material with your name
- Link to pro website
- Professional letter of reference

BH Cosmetics
https://camerareadycosmetics.com/collections/bh-cosmetics

Requirement(s): Apply and Refer to Camera Ready Cosmetics guidelines.

Billion Dollar Brows
http://pro.billiondollarbrows.com/become-a-pro/

Requirement(s); Fill out the online application for pro artist consideration or Contact Billion Dollar Brows at priscilla@billiondollarbrows.com or by phone at 310-247-3227

Black Up Cosmetics
https://www.blackupcosmetics.com

I was unable to verify a pro artist program with Black Up

Cosmetics.

Blinc Collection
https://camereadycosmetics.com/collections/blinc

Requirement(s): Apply and Refer to Camera Ready
Cosmetics guidelines.

Bodyography
https://www.bodyography.com/pages/pro-discount

Requirement(s); Once you have created an account, fill
out the form and submit one of the following:

- Cosmetology License
- Esthetician License
- Certificate from a makeup school/program
- Business Card and or/website address
- Portfolio to show professional makeup work

Fill out the online form and submit your documents.

Calm Skincare
https://www.calmskincare.com/register.asp

Requirement(s); Fill out the online application and submit
the required documents.

Camera Ready Cosmetics
https://camerareadycosmetics.com/pages/pro-makeup-
artist-discount

Requirement(s); Fill out the online application and submit

2 of the following required documents

- Website portfolio
- Call Sheet
- Union ID
- Cosmetology or Esthetician License
- Scan of an editorial submission with your name
- Copy of tax return or liability insurance

Cao Cosmetics
https://caocosmeticsusa.com

I was unable to verify a Pro Artist Program on their website at this time. Check back for this program in the future.

Cara Cosmetics
http://www.caracosmetics.com/pro-discount/

Requirement(s); To apply, completely fill out the form below. If you don't have a website or you're a student, email us a scan of your comp card, a tear sheet (with printed name credit), professional license or diploma, proof of your enrollment or union card.

Email: sales@caracosmetics.com

Cara will contact you with your custom discount code upon approval.

Cargo Cosmetics
http://www.cargocosmetics.com/pro-artist-program/

Apply Online

Requirement(s): a copy of one piece of valid photo identification plus copies of two of the following indicating your current employment as a makeup artist:

- Valid union card
- Makeup artist certificate or professional license
- TV or film crew call list
- Professional letter of reference stating employment
- Editorial page including your credit

Please forward these items along with your email address and mailing address (including postal or ZIP code) to: customerservice@cargocosmetics.com

Or mail to:

TPR Holdings LLC

875 Third Ave, 7th Floor
New York, NY 10022
Please be sure to include all of your contact information.

Please note that The CARGO Pro Artist Program is available only to artists in the United States and Canada. CARGO reserves the right to reject an application or request additional documentation at our discretion

Questions? customerservice@cargocosmetics.com

Cinema Secrets
https://camerareadycosmetics.com/collections/cinema-secrets

Requirement(s): Refer to Camera Ready Cosmetics guidelines.

Colorscience

https://www.colorescience.com/professional-makeup-artists

Requirement(s) Colorescience Professional Artistry Program is currently available in the United States only. The special discounts associated with Colorescience Artistry program are exclusive to Colorescience professionals, and membership is non-transferable. Fill out online application to be considered Requirement(s): website, photo ID, license or certificate.

CoverFX

https://www.coverfx.com

The Professional Makeup Artist program is closed at this time. The website says to check back to their FAQ for pro discounts in the future.

Crown Brush

https://www.crownbrush.com/pages/crown-pro-application

Apply Online
Requirement(s) photo identification, (1) piece of current professional criteria:

- Composite Card
- Editorial page with name credit
- Union Card
- Professional License Diploma/Certificate
- Publication Master Head

- Program/Press Materials w/ Name Contract on Production Master Head
- Program/Press Materials w/ Name
- Contract on Production Letterhead
- Professional Letter of Reference of Employment

Questions? crownpro@crownbrush.com for your application.

Danessa Myricks Beauty
https://camerareadycosmetics.com/collections/danessa-myricks-beauty

Requirement(s): Refer to Camera Ready Cosmetics guidelines.

Dinair Pro Airbrush
https://www.airbrushmakeup.com/pro/

Apply Online

Requirement(s): A copy of photo identification, certificate, resume.

DUO
https://camerareadycosmetics.com/collections/duo

Requirement(s): Refer to Camera Ready Cosmetics guidelines.

Ecco Bella
https://www.eccobella.com/eb-pro/

Apply Online
Requirement(s): Fill out the application form and be sure to attach copies of your valid ID and credentials with the application. Pro's will need to create an account on www.eccobella.com

Ellis Faas
www.ellisfaas.com

Requirement(s) makeup artists, cosmetologists, and aestheticians, hairstylists, nail technicians, models, photographers, Fashion Stylists, Costume Designer, On air performer, & make up student

Embryolisse
https://camerareadycosmetics.com/collections/embryolisse

Requirement(s): Refer to Camera Ready Cosmetics guidelines.

Essie
https://www.essie.com/register/pro

Apply Online
Requirement(s): Professional license: cosmetologist, cosmetologist instructor or nail tech.

European Body Art
https://camerareadycosmetics.com/collections/european-body-art

Requirement(s): Refer to Camera Ready Cosmetics guidelines.

Eve Pearl
https://camareadycosmetics.com/collections/eve-pearl

Requirement(s): Refer to Camera Ready Cosmetics guidelines.

Eye Kandy Cosmetics
https://camareadycosmetics.com/collections/eye-kandy

Requirement(s): Refer to Camera Ready Cosmetics guidelines.

EYEMIMO
http://www.eyemimo.com/makeup-pro/

Requirement(s): Fill out the form on the website, upload business card and submit.

Ey Envy
https://www.eyenvy.ca/contact-wholesale.php

If you are a Salon Owner and would like to carry EyEnvy® in your business, please fill out the online form and include all of your business information. An EyEnvy® customer service representative will get back to you within 48 hours. Office hours are from Monday - Friday from 9am - 5pm Eastern Time. If you need an immediate answer or would like to reach us by telephone please do so by calling our toll free number at 1.888.770.3689

Facade Beauty Makeup
http://www.facadebeauty.com

Apply Online
Requirement(s): Add registration form to our bag and fill
out online. Applications will be approved in 5-10 days.

FACEatelier
https://www.faceatelier.com/proartists/

Apply Online
Requirement(s): two current items from the following list:

- Composite Card Business Card with name and
  specific profession
- Editorial with credit
- Union Card
- Professional License
- Diploma/Certificate
- IMBD link
- Website link
- Video/reel link
- Publication Masthead
- Program/Press Materials with name
- Contract on Production Company Letterhead
- Crew/Call List on Production Company
  Letterhead
- Professional Letter of Reference or Employment

Fashion Fair
http://www.fashionfair.com/pp_form.php

Complete Online Application
Requirement(s): Any two of the following along with
photo identification is required:

- Magazine tear sheet with name credit

- Program or call sheet
- Union membership card
- Proof of agency representation (letter from agent or link to the roster)
- Website (gallery sites or Facebook not valid)
- Blank Contract

Flutter Lashes
https://camareadycosmetics.com/collections/flutter-lashes

Requirement(s): Refer to Camera Ready Cosmetics guidelines.

Fortunate Face Minerals
http://fortunatefaceminerals.com/pro-artist-program/

Requirement(s): Two of the following:

- pro website
- pro business card
- tear sheet
- call sheet
- student ID/State or your license and state

Email your documents to
info@fortunatefaceminerals.com

Once you have been verified you will be issued a pro discount code to use at checkout.

Frankie Rose Cosmetics
http://frankierosecosmetics.com/frankie-pro

Download pro form and complete all requirements then email to: pro@frankierosecosmetics.com
Requirement(s): Two of the following:

- Professional license (cosmetology or esthetician)
- Makeup certificate (80 hours or more)
- Crew/call list on production company letterhead
- Link to website
- Union card
- Business card
- Editorial page with a name credit

Frends Beauty
https://www.frendsbeauty.com/fwb-pro-l-fb.html

Requirement(s): Fill out online application.

Funk n' Frost
https://funknfrost.com/pages/funk-n-frost-pro-membership

Download application
Requirement(s): Two of the following:

- A copy of your business card
- 2 professional letters of reference
- 2 of the latest projects you have worked on
- Your website/online profile
- A copy of a bill or invoice for work completed

Email completed application to: discount@funknfrost.com

FURLESS Cosmetics
https://furlesscosmetics.com/blogs/default-blog/furless-mua-pro-club-application

Apply Online
Requirement(s): To apply, please provide your details below, including your website link. Please note that social media pages such as Facebook pages, Instagram, or Model Mayhem pages will not be accepted as a website. A dedicated website with your business contact details as well as your portfolio will be required.

Fusion Of Color
https://www.fusionofcolor.net/PRO-DISCOUNT.html

Apply Online
Requirement(s): To apply, email a link to your website or online portfolio, along with your mailing address, phone number and preferred email address. If you do not have a website, send us a scan of your comp card, a tear sheet (with printed name credit), professional license, diploma or union card instead. Still a student of makeup artistry or cosmetology? You must register an account before applying. When we receive your credentials, then we will change you to a PRO account. E-mail all information to pro@fusionofcolor.net

Gorgeous Cosmetics
https://gorgeouscosmetics.com/pages/gorgeous-pro-program

Requirement(s): complete online application
- Business card with name and specific profession
- Call sheet on production company letterhead

- Composite card (models only)
- Contract on production company letterhead
- Professional letter of employment or pay stub from client, salon manager, or cosmetic retailer
- Professional license, diploma/certificate
- Professional website (social media sites not accepted)
- Program or press materials with name
- Publication masthead
- Tear sheet with name credit
- Union card
- Headshot (for models and actors only)

Illamasqua
https://www.illamasqua.com

Apply Online
Requirement(s):
- Website link (not social media)
- Business insurance certificate (must be for the beauty industry)
- BABTEC Membership
- Certificate/diploma from full-time school of makeup artistry (minimum 50 hours)
- Call sheet (full LTD company address)
- BECTU Membership with ID card (makeup and hair branch)
- BAFTA Member ship with ID card
- Nasmah Member
- Proof of agency representation (name listed on agency website)
- Program or press material (must include name and profession)
- Tutor college badge

- Tutor post graduate certificate in education (PGCE)

Inglot
https://inglotcosmetics.com
Apply Online
Requirement(s):
- Pro Membership Card from other approved Makeup Programs
- License of accredited schools of cosmetics
- Magazine tear sheet with name credit
- Real with name credit
- Program/call sheet
- Union Membership Card
- Makeup Artist Business Card
- Agency Representation
- Student ID or Enrollment Documentation
- Professional Headshot

It Cosmetics
https://www.itcosmetics.com/proshow

Apply Online
Requirement(s): Professional applicants must provide a valid photo ID and 2 professional credentials from within the last 2 years. One of the professional credentials must be a union card, agency comp card, professional license, or current letter of employment. The other may be a union card, agency comp card, professional license, diploma or certificate from an accredited makeup or cosmetology school, editorial page with name credit, call sheet on production company letterhead, tear sheet with name credit, letter of employment or paystub from a client, salon

or cosmetics retailer, or a professional website.

Jouer Cosmetics
https://www.jouercosmetics.com

Apply Online
Requirement(s): Create an account and apply

Kaia Naturals
https://kaianaturals.com/makeup-artist-program/

Email the following to info@kaianaturals.com
Requirement(s): A copy of your resume and (2) examples
of professional identification that include one of the
following: union card, professional license or publication
masthead, or any two of the following:

- composite card
- editorial page with name credit
- program or press material with name and
  profession
- contract on professional letterhead
- professional website
- professional letter of reference of employment
- and/or certificate/ diploma

Required professional identification must be current
(within one year) and indicate your name and specific
profession.

Kat Von D
https://www.katvondbeauty.com/pro-application

Requirement(s): Apply Online: Submit a photo or scan of
your valid government-issued photo ID and ONE current
credential from the list below:

- IATSE Union card
- Professional license (for aestheticians, cosmetologists or salon makeup artists)
- Publication masthead

OR submit a photo or scan of your valid government-issued photo ID and TWO current credentials from the list below:

- Agency branded composite card
- Certificate/diploma from full-time school of makeup artistry (minimum of 90 hrs.)
- Editorial page with name credit (must include date within the last 12 months)
- Program or press material (must include name, profession and date within the last 12 months)
- Self-hosted professional website (not social media)
- Proof of agency representation (listed on agencies' website)
- Call sheet on product company letterhead (must include date within the last 12 months)
- Paystub noting profession (must include date within the last 12 months)

Kett Cosmetics
https://www.kettcosmetics.com/wholesale-registration-page/

Apply Online
Requirement(s): Two of the following:

- Hair or Makeup Union Card
- Cosmetology or Esthetician License
- Tear Sheet with credit
- Film or commercial call sheet

- An on-line portfolio link with makeup images

Kevin Aucoin
https://kevynaucoinbeauty.com/pages/pro-artist-registration

Apply Online
Requirement(s): Professional Makeup Artists, Aesthetician Cosmetologist. Create an account on the website

Koh Gen Do
https://kohgendocosmetics.com/pages/beauty-pro
Apply Online

Requirement(s): Fill out the online form and submit required information.

Kryolan
https://us.kryolan.com/procard/about

Apply Online
Requirement(s): Fill out the request form and provide proof that you are a working professional in the hair and/or makeup industry

Lashes In A Box
https://www.lashesinabox.com

Requirement(s): Fill out the request form and provide proof that you are a working professional in the hair and/or makeup industry

Laura Geller
https://www.laurageller.com/professional-program

Apply Online
Requirement(s):
You must submit a copy of your valid photo ID. AND
You must submit two of the following for consideration:

- business card.
- current agency ZED card OR comp card.
- professional license.
- professional resume.
- two professional tear sheets with your name credited.
- valid union card.

Laura Mercier
https://www.lauramercier.com/professional-artist-program.html

Requirement(s): *Agency Representation: Have agency fax a roster list on company letterhead or provide link to agency website *Film or Television Experience: Fax crew list with name credited as a makeup artist on set.*Tear sheets with name credit *Copy of your Union Card (Drivers Licenses, Business Cards and Educational Certificates are NOT acceptable forms of ID) send this information to the attention of Professional Makeup Artist Program at our email address of makeup.artists@lauramercier.com

Le Cosmétique
https://www.lacosmetique.com.au

Requirement(s): A link to your website, blog or online

portfolio, Makeup Artist Training Certificate, Copy of your cosmetology/esthetics license, Comp Card or Tear Sheet (with credit)

London Brush Company
https://sianrichardslondon.com/srl-pro/

Apply Online
Requirement(s): A copy of your Photo ID & One of the following: Website, IMDB Page, Union Card, Call Sheet

LORAC (through Naime's)
https://www.naimies.com/studio-pro-invitation.php

Request an application online using the website link above.
Requirement(s):You will need to contact the NAIME'S NAIME'S Beauty Center • naimes.com • 12640 Riverside Drive, Valley Village, CA 91607 • 818.655.9933

Lotus Lashes
https://www.lotuslashes.com/pages/be-a-lotus-pro

Apply Online
Requirement(s): Upload Resume and/or Professional License, Diploma/Certificate

Makeup Artist Network
http://www.makeupart.net

Apply Online
Requirement(s): submit (2) two pieces of professional identification

Make Up For Ever
https://www.makeupforever.com/us/en-us/pro-only

Apply online
Requirement(s): Makeup Artist – Open to all working
professional makeup artists

The Makeup Light
https://themakeuplight.com/pages/artist-relations

Apply Online
Requirement: Fill out form on website

Mally Cosmetics
www.mallybeauty.com

Apply Online
Requirement(s): Submit proof that you are a currently
working Artist, cosmetician, or other makeup professional.

Mecca Cosmetica
https://www.mecca.com.au/beauty-loop.html

Requirement(s): If you would like to apply, please contact
Customer Service team via email
customerservice@mecca.com.au and we will email you an
application form.

Mehron
https://www.mehron.com/all-pro-discounts/

Requirement(s): Must be a pro member of: The Power

Group, Professional Beauty Association (PBA), Or Make-Up Magazine. See chapter three to learn the details on how to apply to these professional organizations.

Mirabella Beauty
https://www.mirabellabeauty.com/pages/professionals

Apply Online
Requirement(s):

- photo ID
- valid business license
- state certification
- other documentation that demonstrates your application as an industry professional

Motives Cosmetics
https://www.motivescosmetics.com/join/pro-artist

Apply Online
Requirement(s): a copy of your photo identification, and examples of your work to the address listed on the application.

Morphe Brushes
https://www.morphebrushes.com/collections/pro-memberships

Apply Online
Requirement(s): Graduate from a professional beauty program: Certificate of completion (makeup program) OR Cosmetology/Esthetician license, Photocopy of ID
Self taught makeup artist: Copy of your business card, Link to your website.

Muse Beauty
https://musebeauty.pro/pro-discount-program/

Apply Online
Requirement(s):

- Agency Composite Card
- Business Card with Name and Specific Profession
- Editorial Page with Name Credit
- Union Card Crew/Call List on Production Company Letterhead
- Professional Letter of Representation on Agency Letterhead
- The Powder Group Pro Membership Card

MUD (Makeup-Up Designatory)
http://www.makeupdesignory.com

Requirement(s): fill out the online form and submit

NARS Cosmetics
https://www.narscosmetics.com/USA/artist-program.html

Apply Online
Requirement(s): application and professional proof

Naked Cosmetics
http://nakedcosmetics.com/proartist/

Apply Online
Requirement(s): All Pro Make-Up Artists, Cosmetologists,

Estheticians, Beauty Students in School, Nail Techs, Hair Stylists, Performers, Models, On-Air Personalities, Designers, Photographers, and other Industry Professionals may apply.

Napoleon Perdis
https://napoleonperdis.com/aus/contact_us

Requirement(s): qualification certificates, business card, licenses, press clippings, media advertisements.

Nigel Beauty
https://www.nigelbeauty.com/t-pro.aspx

Requirement(s):

- School Diploma
- Valid Cosmetology or Esthetician license
- Tear Sheet With Name Credit
- Dedicated Website Promoting Work
- Pro Membership Card, Invoice/Proof of Professional Work, Agency Comp Card
- Valid Union Card or Program or Call Sheet

NYX Cosmetics
https://www.nyxcosmetics.com/proregister

Apply Online
Requirement(s): a copy of your Photo ID plus Option A – a copy of your active cosmetology license/certificate Option B – a copy of your business card, 3 trade references, 3 of the latest projects you have worked on or your website/online profile, and a copy of a bill or invoice for work. If submitting tear sheets, your name must be credited.

Norcostco Cosmetics
https://www.norcostco.com/makeup-cl.aspx

Apply Online
Requirement(s): a business card or a copy of your license

Nudestix
https://www.nudestix.com/pages/pro-page

Apply Online
Requirement(s): Fill out request form and provide proof that you are a working professional in the hair and/or makeup industry

OPI
www.opi.com

Requirement(s): Professional license – cosmetologist, cosmetologist instructor or nail tech.

Origins Skincare
https://www.origins.com/account/

Apply Online

Paint And Powder Store
https://www.paintandpowderstore.com/artistdiscount.php

Apply Online
Requirement(s): Registration form and copy of your ID, you must also include a copy of (1) of the qualifying

documents below:

- Union ID Card
- Agency Comp Card
- Copy of a valid State Board issued Cosmetology or Esthetician license
- Your IMDB Link with credits as a makeup or hair stylist
- Call sheet issued by a production company for a paid job, dated within the last 12 months
- Published magazine editorial tear sheet with your name

Paula Dorf
https://www.pauladorf.com/faq

Requirement(s): Provide at least two forms of ID.
Agency Representation: Fax a roster list on company letterhead Film or Television Experience:
Fax crew list with production name Freelance Makeup Artist

Please provide at least two of the following:
Crew list, Letterhead with production company name, Call Sheets or Tear sheets, Copy of a Union Card, Resume (A Drivers License is NOT an acceptable form of ID)

Submit to:

Professional Makeup Artist Program
Paula Dorf Cosmetics
c/o PDR
110 Fieldcrest Avenue, Suite 23
Edison, NJ 08837
Fax: 732-313-4437

ColourPop
https://colourpop.com/pages/students

Student Discount
Requirement(s): Fill out request form and provide proof
that you are a working professional in the hair and/or
makeup industry

Royal & Langnickel
https://beautyusa.royalbrush.com

Apply Online
Requirement(s): Fill out form

Sally Beauty
In Person Application Required
Requirement(s): Bring professional beauty license or proof
of salon ownership and complete the application to your
local Sally Beauty Supply store

Senna Cosmetics
https://sennacosmetics.com/senna-pro-benefits/

Apply Online
Requirement(s): Complete online application with all
required documents attached.

Serenity + Scott Beauty
https://shop.serenityscottbeauty.com/pro-contact/

Apply Online
Requirement(s): fill out form

Shue Uemura
https://www.shuuemura-usa.com

Requirement(s): Create an account and fill out information

Sigma Beauty
https://www.sigmabeauty.com/sigma-pro

Apply Online
Requirement(s): Driver's license or state/federal photo ID
& One of the following:

- Professional website
- Call list on production company letterhead
- Editorial Page and publication cover dated within the last six months
- Professional license (cosmetology, aesthetician)
- Union Card or IMDB Credit

Smashbox
https://www.smashbox.com/smashbox-pro

Apply Online
Requirement(s): All three levels require valid ID

- drivers license
- certificate program verification (freelance)
- valid cosmetology or esthetician license
- professional letter of reference (pro)

Spectrum Cosmetics
https://www.spectrumcollections.com/pages/pro-artist

Apply Online

Requirement(s): Two of the following:

- Professional license
- business card
- professional website
- tear sheet with real name
- valid union card
- comp card
- letter of employment

Stila Cosmetics
https://www.stilacosmetics.com/the-pro-artist-program.html

Download Application and submit via email to proartist@stilacosmetics.com

Requirement(s): Two of the following:

- composite card
- portfolio with name credit
- business card
- valid union card
- head shot
- publication masthead
- professional license/diploma
- program/press materials with name credit
- contract on production company letterhead
- crew/call list on production company letterhead
- professional letter of reference company letterhead

Studio Gear Cosmetics
https://studiogearcosmetics.com/pages/pro-artists

Please submit application information to the attention of:
Professional Makeup Artist Program
Email: support@studiogearcosmetics.com
Mail: 400 South Avenue, Suite 2, Middlesex, NJ 08846
Fax: 732-868-3055
Requirement(s): two of the following:

- agency representation or provide a
- link to the agency web site,
- Film or Television Experience
- Crew list with name credit
- Tear sheets with name credit
- Copy of your Union Card

Drivers Licenses, Business Cards and Education
Certificates are NOT acceptable forms of ID.

Tarte
www.tartecosmetics.com

As of September 7, 2017, Tarte is accepting applications
via email. Please send the following application elements
to info@tarte.com. They will review your application and
respond to you within a 2-3 weeks.
Application Requirements:
- Valid license or form of identification
- Copy of valid artist certification
- Copy of resume
- Email address

Temptu

https://temptu.com/pro/frequently-asked-questions

Submit the following via email

Requirement(s): Tear Sheet w/Name Credit, Agency Comp Card, Valid Union Card, Crew/Call Sheet with Name Credit, Valid Cosmetology or Esthetician License, Letter of Employment

The Perfect Face
https://www.tpfcosmetics.com/pages/pro-artist-program

Requirement(s): proof of your profession such as business cards, state license etc.

Three Custom Colors
www.threecustom.com

Call to register for their pro artist program

Urban Decay
https://www.urbandecay.com/udpro

Requirement(s): A copy of your driver 's license or state/federal photo ID. Two of the following: Professional license (cosmetology), Editorial page with name credit, Crew/call list on production company letterhead, Union card, Link to website, Business Card or Professional letter of reference

Velour Lashes

https://www.velourlashes.com

Requirement(s): Fill out application and submit proof of professional documentation.

Viseart Paris
https://www.viseartparis.com/pro-signup

Submit the following information to pro@viseartparis.com for consideration: Photo ID along with two of the following:
- School Transcript
- Call Sheet
- Tear Sheet
- Contract
- Deal Memo
- Professional License or Certificate
- Proof of LLC
- Professional Website
- Agency Representation
- Credited Editorial Shoot
- Active Union Card

Yaby Cosmetics
https://yabycosmetics.com/pages/industry-discount-application

Requirement(s): one of the following documents in a single PDF file:

- Call Sheet
- Editorial Credits
- Union Membership Card

- Professional Reference Letter
- Proof of registration with photo ID (for students who are currently in a cosmetics or aesthetics program)
- Cosmetics or aesthetics certificate/diploma with photo ID (dated within last 12 months)

Zuca
https://www.zuca.com/business-and-beauty

Email: customerservice@zuca.com
Requirement(s): Fill out the form found at the link above to be sent the application to submit professional content.

PROFESSIONAL ORGANIZATIONS

Like any career industry, it is essential to join professional associations in the beauty industry to get ahead and network with like-minded people. Whether you are a beauty industry student, aspiring makeup artist, or a freelance professional, you should have a network of people who can connect you to opportunities. Networking should become a purposeful part of your career, and you should always be prepared to seize the moment.

Here are three professional organizations you can join today and start your career off as a member of an organization that can keep you informed and in touch with your industry and today's industry standards.

Professional Beauty Association

The Professional Beauty Association (PBA) is a non-profit that exists to elevate, unite and serve the beauty industry and the professionals who improve people's lives.

Learn more about the benefits of becoming a Member!

https://probeauty.org/join/

The Powder Group

From coast to coast and around the world The Powder Group brings artists together like never before while providing access to the most relevant makeup industry information, career guidance, promotional opportunities, and the biggest artists, brands and products in the makeup business. The Powder Group invites you become a part of the fastest growing artist community anywhere, and we are thrilled to announce the new TPG Pro Membership program.

Participation in the program affords you a wide variety of members only benefits to help to keep you inspired, informed and motivated, they benefits that will help you grow you as an artist, strengthen your relationships, and deepen your connection to the artist industry.

Join The Powder Group and see what membership can mean to you and your career.

Apply Online

http://www.thepowdergroup.com/index.html

Make-Up Magazine

Make-Up Artist magazine is thrilled to partner with many makeup brands offering discounts at IMATS. The *Make-Up Artist* magazine Pro Card is recognized by Kat Von D, M·A·C Cosmetics, Make Up For Ever and NARS as setting an industry standard vetting credentials for makeup artists worldwide. Your Pro Card gives you access to their pro discounts year-round. Their list of cosmetic companies is continuing to grow as they strive to bring more to the community they serve.

Apply Online

https://makeupmag.com/pro/pro-credentials

YOUR PRO CARD JOURNAL

Use this journal to keep track of your pro cards, website links, login information, and your passwords. You may be required to re-apply annually or bi-annually, be sure to note that on your journal entry.

1.

2.

3.

4.

5.

6.

7.

8.

9.

10.

11.

12.

13.

14.

15.

16.

17.

18.

19.

20.

21.

22.

23.

24.

25.

26.

27.

28.

29.

30.

31.

32.

33.

34.

35.

36.

37.

38.

39.

40.

41.

42.

43.

44.

45.

46.

47.

48.

49.

50.

ABOUT THE AUTHOR

Toni Thomas is an award-winning beauty industry professional, New York Fashion Week and editorial makeup artist, beauty educator, and author of several beauty industry books. Her makeup artistry has been featured in many fashion publications and she can be found twice a year at New York Fashion Week. Toni is the founder of Women in Gear, The School of Makeup Artistry an online education portal for aspiring makeup artists. Toni has spent her entire career in the beauty industry working in and around the beauty business as well as the beauty education arena where she has taught for many years. Opening her first salon in 1993 she proved that even young women can and will conquer the world of business and she has been an independent small business owner ever since.

Today you can find her working hard on a new book or on location doing fashion photo shoots, she also works as a consultant giving guidance to some of today's trendiest salons and spas! She has committed her life to her passion in the beauty business, teaching in the world of beauty to those who are willing to take a leap of faith on themselves, and it is what she aspires to do the rest of her life. As one of the pioneers for quality online education, she is committed to all aspects of an industry that has lacked credibility for far too long and she is committed to teaching women across the globe how to build their beauty businesses with passion and patience.

Born and raised in Montana, she now travels with her husband between their home in the mountains of Montana and their home on the lake in Virginia. Her passion to inspire has made a global impact on the world of business, makeup, and beauty.

The following list of books she has authored can be found on Amazon.com:

<u>THE BUSINESS OF MAKEUP ARTISTRY: Your Guide to a Successful Beauty Business</u>

<u>DIY BRIDAL MAKEUP: 10 Steps to Flawless Wedding Day Makeup</u>

<u>MAKEUP MAGIC: A Pocket Guide to Flawless Everyday Makeup</u>

<u>PROFESSIONAL MAKEUP ARTISTRY: A Five Star Guide to Professional Makeup</u>

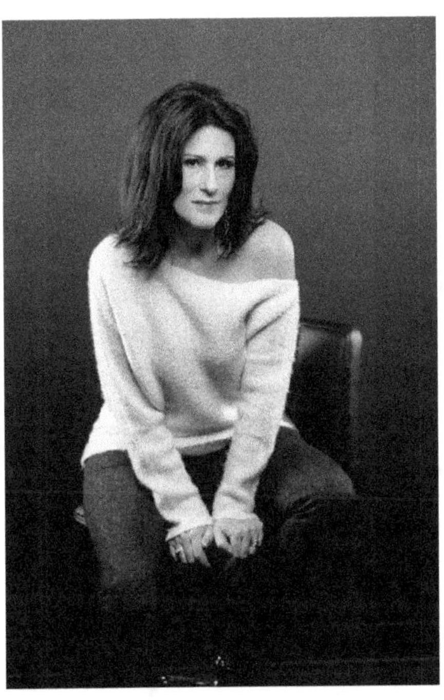

You can follow her work and upcoming events at:

Toni Thomas, The American Makeup Artist
www.theamericanmakeupartist.com
Instagram: @toni_thomas_mua
Facebook: @tonithomasmua